CURING THE BODY OFF DEPRESSION AND ANXIETY

EASY STEPS TO OVERCOME DEPRESSION AND ANXIETY

BY

DR AMANDA F. LOPEZ

Table of Contents

PREFACE

Why did I write this book and who I am?

I am a naturopathic physician who specializes in gestalt therapy, a type of psychotherapy. Counseling and improving people's physical health are two ways I assist a lot of people with emotional issues. Because, as you've probably noticed, people with physical and emotional problems have a very difficult time getting better, my job is both satisfying and frustrating.

Some people take a lot of medications and herbal and nutritional supplements, but they never get over their emotional problems. Others seek counseling or read books on cultivating a positive mindset, but never experience physical healing. Because it is necessary to heal your mind and body simultaneously in order to fully recover, this book shows you how to combine holistic medicine with positive thinking.

This book combines my own personal experience with tried-and-true treatments I use with my patients to treat a wide range of emotional issues, including sadness, emotional pain, depression, anxiety, fear, irritability, stress, dissatisfaction, fatigue, and others. Both I and many of my patients, who are now happier and more emotionally stable, have benefited from these methods.

Even though emotional well-being is the main focus of this book, if you follow my advice, you can get rid of a lot of other problems, like digestive issues, hormonal issues, skin issues, obesity, asthma, joint problems, and other chronic diseases. This is because this book focuses a lot on reducing inflammation, stress, and imbalance in your body, which are the main causes of most chronic diseases.

This book will teach you the following.

This book explains the various factors that influence your emotions. You will discover how your emotional experiences are influenced by physical factors. I'll show you how upsetting encounters affect profound prosperity and I give you strong mental procedures to recuperate from pressure and difficult profound encounters. In order to become more emotionally resilient and remain well for longer, you will learn how to resolve turbulent emotions, change negative thoughts and beliefs, rewire your brain, and develop more positive thoughts and habits.

This book is written for anyone who wants to feel better, even though I use the terms anxiety and depression a lot. Anyone who wants to reduce stress, recover from stressful experiences in the past, or simply feel more energized, healthy, and optimistic can benefit from the advice in this book. We all go through challenging times in our lives that necessitate healing.

Sadly, surveys reveal that the stigma associated with emotional issues prevents many people from seeking treatment or even admitting they have a problem. Despite the fact that they have a condition that is very treatable and results from very reasonable and non-shameful causes, some people fear that they will be judged as weak or incapable of coping with life. Some people avoid seeking assistance because they believe that their depressed feelings are inherent to their personality. Sadly, many of these individuals fail to seek assistance and allow their lives to continue to deteriorate, sometimes even to the point of suicide.

This book is not meant to take the place of professional medical advice. My objective is to assist you in treating the underlying causes of your emotional problems, to resolve unresolved emotional experiences that contribute to your current emotional state, and to enable you to make better choices on the path to well-being. I additionally trust that therapists will peruse this book and look past simple drugs to help individuals feel quite a bit improved. If you use the methods in this book, you might find that you need less medication. Before attempting any of the treatments described here or altering any of your medications, please exercise caution and seek the advice of a qualified professional.

<u>INTRODUCTION</u>

Knowing which kind of person has a disease is more important

"My wellbeing was not equivalent to it was previously, I could feel it. Far more atrocious, my feelings were winding up in a very difficult situation. I would lie in bed or on the floor, once in a while crying unnecessarily and having sympathy for myself. Crying would some way or another bring me help, yet the despair won't ever move. I didn't feel energetic any longer. I had no inspiration or certainty to do new things. My energy dislike it used to be. What I used to appreciate in the past didn't feel like such a lot of fun any longer. Was there a major issue with me? What was off-base with me? What had transformed me? I felt off-kilter conversing with specific individuals since I figured they wouldn't really care for me. I likewise felt remorseful without any problem. For what reason did I feel so remorseful? I needed to conceal my tears in some cases while strolling in the roads… tears of profound torment for now and then obscure reasons. Had somebody let me know I was discouraged, I would have opposed, since I realized I was a more grounded individual, and as I would like to think discouraged individuals required meds and I questioned I wanted medicine. I just needed to sort out some way to escape this state… "

Do any of these sentiments sound natural to you? They could not. Despite the fact that I could do without to just own it, this was me, battling with declining wellbeing and sentiments of trouble, uneasiness, and conceivable sorrow after a long distressing period in my life. Fortunately, in light of my preparation and huge assistance from my partners, I gotten myself away from this foreboding shadow. Utilizing the strategies I have portrayed in this book, I can genuinely say that I am a lot better and more joyful now; I feel more persuaded, lighter, secure with myself; and I have a lot better private connections. I currently even run preparing workshops, profound mending and group building studios and wellbeing withdraws in extraordinary areas in Africa.

<u>FACTORS THAT HAVE AN IMPACT ON MENTAL HEALTH</u>

Despite the fact that I was battling sincerely with a tough spot in my life, I immediately acknowledged it was not just outside encounters that were influencing my prosperity. The things I ate and my movement levels were emphatically affecting my psychological and actual wellbeing. I was truly defenseless against medical problems, weariness, tension and burdensome contemplations. It was shortly after I begun changing my eating regimen and way of life, practicing and taking spices and enhancements that I started to understand the solid physiological association with my feelings. My way of life propensities were significantly affecting my body's science and my body's science was straightforwardly influencing my mind science. I likewise worked with different specialists to discharge close to home encounters from before, which were influencing the way I taken a gander at the world and impeding me from partaking in my current life.

As a result of my own insight, my preparation, and involvement in various patients, I truly believe you should take a gander at the accompanying parts of your life in the event that you are battling with medical conditions or your feelings and are attempting to acquire profound harmony and strength:

1. Has there been any actually or sincerely horrendous mishap in your life?

On the off chance that there has been close to home injury or upsetting occasions in your day to day existence, the limbic piece of your mind stays focused even a long time after the injury, and an oblivious piece of you never completely recuperates. You wind up carrying on with life forever impacted by the occasion. It turns into a piece of your story. Treatments like guiding, psychotherapy, homeopathic drugs, or Bach bloom cures, all of which I examine in later parts, assist with setting profound injury free from your cognizant and oblivious brain and from your limbic mind. By delivering close to home injury, you start to encounter life from a position of solidarity, energy, and genuineness.

2. Is a natural or synthetic unevenness influencing your feelings?

Your psyche is impacted by synapses, chemicals, and other compound couriers drifting around your body. Synapses and chemicals are straightforwardly impacted by supplements in the food varieties you eat, ecological poisons, and furthermore by the wellbeing of your various organs. In the following parts, you will figure out how your liver, adrenal organs, thyroid organ, and stomach related framework influence your state of mind. You will likewise figure out how to recuperate these organs and utilize the right food varieties, supplements, and spices to address the equilibrium of your body. Doing this will improve your prosperity with durable outcomes, and decrease the ups what's more, downs many individuals go through when they depend just on impermanent fixes

3. Is there an upsetting circumstance in your life or a direction for living that is obstructing your capacity to mend?

Constant pressure is the quickest method for breaking an individual. Being around basic, forceful, or genuinely harmful individuals keeps you in an unending condition of stress. On the off chance that you are in an upsetting circumstance, whether socially or at work, you need to remove quick moves toward move from it or look for help to adapt to it in a better and more enabled way. Similarly, you really want to work out routinely to assist your body with recuperating from pressure and figure out how to stay away from certain undesirable exercises. Ordinary exercises that you might believe are helping you unwind can really worsen your feelings of anxiety. Things like drinking as well much liquor or observing a lot of television disrupt your possibilities of recuperating completely. Manhandling opiate drugs, chattering about others, talking adversely about existence, spending time with individuals who don't advance your prosperity, investing an excessive amount of energy at work without really focusing on yourself, and doing things that don't assist you with feeling better are likewise ways you stress your mind and your body without knowing it.

Pointless and unfortunate propensities disrupt close to home mending and take up important time that could be spent working on your wellbeing. Attempt and fill each extra second or inactive time you have in the day with better exercises, like activity, positive discussions, perusing moving books, yoga, reflection, breathing activities, and social exercises that improve your sense of prosperity instead of make you wiped out and frustrated later on. In later sections, I show you some simple lighthearted activities you can do to top off your day and recuperate your feelings.

"Jane" was a 34 year-old patient of mine experiencing ongoing discouragement. She had been a worker in Somalia and had experienced distressing contentions with her partners. She experienced sleep deprivation and gorging as a component of her downturn. She had likewise experienced persistent cerebral pains since she was a youngster and had encountered her dad being oppressive toward her mom when she was growing up. The profound injury of her experience growing up had left her inclination powerless during clashes, which drove her to move in an opposite direction from defending herself as a grown-up and expanded her pressure at work.

For Jane's situation, her profound family ancestry assumed a gigantic part in her helplessness to dread and gloom. Simultaneously, her ongoing pressure had drained her adrenal organs (adrenal organ wellbeing is shrouded broadly in impending sections), leaving her depleted and incapable to defeat profound issues. What's more, her gorging of a great deal of bland food varieties, joined with her stress, caused her glucose, cortisol, and insulin levels to become unsound, leaving her exasperated and inclined to compound uneven characters that impacted her state of mind and her wellbeing. As a feature of Jane's mending process, we urged her to eat good food varieties, which worked fair and square of cerebrum synthetic compounds in her blood. We settled large numbers of her past close to home injuries utilizing psychotherapy and energy based medications (homeopathic and Bach blossom cures, talked about in later sections), assisting her with delivering the horrible encounters that were still impacting her oblivious psyche and influencing her way of behaving. We likewise developed her adrenal organ wellbeing utilizing spices and wholesome enhancements so her synthetic uneven characters were additionally adjusted and balanced out for longer times of time.

Jane's case was a regular instance of sorrow that was settled utilizing a multi- point, complete comprehensive methodology. She needed to address her profound history, her eating regimen, as well as her actual wellbeing to feel sincerely well for longer timeframes.

The methodology of settling close to home encounters, reestablishing your body's ideal actual state and taking part in sound everyday exercises is the foundation of developing an establishment for profound fortitude. By mending the underlying driver, you don't stifle side effects, are less reliant upon medicine, and you will probably feel improved any more timeframes.

THE IMPACTS OF PROFOUND ENCOUNTERS

All profound encounters start a physiological cycle in your body. For each demonstration, feeling, and articulation of adoration, confidence, self-pardoning, and absolution toward another, your body reconnects toward one more physiological cycle, nearer to its unique interaction, its best cycle…

Profound AND Horrendous mishaps affect our wellbeing, be it a relationship separation, guardians battling, divorces, a huge misfortune, monetary troubles, passing of a friend or family member, or another component. Organically talking, your mind can make new brain associations in view of what you experience. This capacity is the very thing that specialists call brain adaptability critical occasions adjust the brain connections in our mind, making new nerve associations be shaped to adapt to the pressure and to expect comparable occasions that may happen from here on out. These new brain associations adjust your view of the world and of yourself so things don't seem equivalent to they used to be the point at which you were dynamic and blissful. These new brain connections likewise change the whole physiology of your body, making organs capability distinctively and causing synthetic compounds, catalysts, and chemicals to be made in various sums, the two of which straightforwardly influence your wellbeing and frustrate your capacity to recuperate genuinely

At times you probably won't actually know that a specific profound occasion has such a significant impact on you. Whenever left unsettled or concealed under a stone in your sub-conscience, the impacts of these encounters keep on influencing your brain and your body deliberately, subliminally, or unwittingly. This makes what I call close to home brief delays, or EHPs, where your brain and body stay impacted and keep on answering close to home encounters as though they were all the while happening, despite the fact that they could have wrapped up. I trust that when the feelings encompassing your experience are excessively enormous for your brain to adapt with, or on the other hand on the off chance that the EHPs happen for a really long time, a piece of your psyche closes somewhere near going into sadness to moderate energy for anticipated encounters. Gloom is likewise halfway because of an absence of confidence in your current circumstance in view of past distressing encounters and is additionally a condition of fatigue your body comes to when it can never again adapt to pressure.

The persistent pressure from EHPs charges your pressure adjusting organs, for example, your adrenal organs and thyroid organs. Overemphasized and under-working adrenal organs are a main source of ongoing tension, misery, and other medical conditions. You really want to determine or release EHPs to address the modified brain processes made in your cerebrum, stop their adverse consequence on your body, and to give your mind a rest, instead of allowed it to stay focused from past occasions. Settling pressure and EHPs is likewise significant on the grounds that genuinely focused organs in your body go through a lot a larger number of supplements and produce a greater number of poisons than in a without a care in the world body. At the point when supplements start to run out in your body, your mind and different organs never again have an adequate number of synapses and chemicals to keep you cheerful and solid.

"John" was thirty years of age and had bipolar confusion, where he vacillated among wretchedness and hyper or hyperactive and restless states. The main driver of his condition was a horrible separation between his folks when he was seven years old and an unsteady home climate while he was growing up. Since he encountered persistent pressure as a small kid, his entire improvement from youth to adulthood was that of a focused on individual. The steady danger and unsteadiness passed at the forefront of his thoughts no real way to have a good sense of security, and he started to foster adapting instruments that were useless to his body's normal cadence.

John's treatment included settling the close to home agony from his recollections utilizing psychotherapy and homeopathic prescriptions and furthermore settling his adrenal organs, which were out of funds receivable to the ongoing tension he grew up with (we will cover homeopathic prescriptions and adrenal organs in later parts). With advising, he understood how much pressure he actually conveyed because of his stressed adolescence. With advising, he likewise fostered the mindfulness and the ability to manage his tension and rethink his grown-up environmental elements with not so much pressure but rather more harmony. He felt more secure confiding in his outside climate. After a couple of meetings of guiding and naturopathic medication, John's condition totally settled, and he had not any more hyper episodes. This was on the grounds that he recuperated his body, yet figured out how to determine his profound brief delays.

Adverse occasions from your past prevent your genuine articulation and adjust the manner in which you associate with others. As you keep on carrying on with your life in a repaid way, you sustain the gloomy sentiments you convey with you. Profound mending is a valuable chance to stir the better and more joyful self-inside you and connect with others and with the world in a more certain manner that definitely gives you more sure encounters. As you recuperate sincerely from previous occasions, you will start to feel more certain and open in your life. With better wellbeing, you can gift yourself a more engaged and positive life.

Releasing and settling pressure and EHPs is conceivable through directing, psychotherapy, conversing with a companion, settling the contention and pardoning. Some of the best treatments I've encountered which discharge EHPs incorporate gestalt treatment, neuron-phonetic programming (NLP), close to home opportunity method (EFT), eye development desensitization and going back over (EMDR, a sort of psychotherapy), contemplation and other psyche body strategies, which I cover in later sections.

Homeopathic medications and Bach bloom cures, canvassed in their own separate sections, are enthusiastic drugs that are likewise extremely viable in settling EHPs.

HOW YOUR ACTUAL BODY INFLUENCES PROFOUND WELLBEING

"To keep the body healthy is an obligation… if not we will not have the option to keep our psyche solid and clear."

I Invested a Ton of energy going for psychotherapy and profound mending with various specialists. Everything functioned admirably; be that as it may, there was dependably a basic uneasiness in my feelings. It was just when I began working out consistently, treating myself with healthful enhancements and ate food varieties that were great for me that I started to see extremely durable outcomes with my profound strength.

Close to home illness is frequently because of an awkwardness of synthetic substances (synapses) in your body and in your mind. The vast majority accept that profound issues are due exclusively to synthetic uneven characters in the cerebrum. Synapses, be that as it may, are created and adjusted by numerous organs in your body, not just your mind, and temperament changes are much of the time a sign of something wrong occurring with one of your different organs.

"Helen" came to see me with a sleeping disorder, nervousness, and excruciating and unpredictable feminine periods. She was having an excessive amount of sugar and drank three cups of espresso daily. The espresso was obstructing her liver capability, which was influencing her rest and her chemicals (I make sense of favoring this in the section "Your

Liver and Close to home Prosperity"). The sugar and espresso were additionally lessening her warm hearted synapses by demolishing her adrenal organs and stomach related framework, which I make sense of in later parts. Her absence of rest was leaving her depleted furthermore, aggravating her tension. She ate not very many vegetables, which starved her group of good supplements and harmed her stomach related framework further, making her wellbeing far more detestable.

We changed her eating routine by eliminating espresso and sugar, and expanding vegetables also, protein-rich food varieties like fish and chicken. We purified her liver utilizing spices and different techniques depicted later in this book. The outcomes were shocking. Her feminine periods became normal, her feminine agonies vanished totally, her nervousness evaporated, and solid rest designs returned in three weeks or less. Not just that, her energy levels and focus improved immensely, and she was given an advancement at work. Her head throbs, which she hadn't drawn out into the open, had likewise evaporated. This is accomplishing ideal wellbeing. Working on your eating routine and reestablishing your organ wellbeing can have astonishing advantages in your day to day existence.

"We should go to nature itself, to the perceptions of the body in wellbeing and in illness to gain proficiency with reality."

~ Hippocrates

The organs separated from your cerebrum that assume a fundamental part in profound solidness are your adrenal organs thyroid organ stomach related framework, and liver. These organ frameworks are additionally pivotal to the groundwork of your general wellbeing. Keeping them sound forestalls and treats numerous different illnesses, including joint inflammation, hormonal awkward nature, ovarian blisters, fibroids, asthma, dermatitis, stomach related issues, and a few other ongoing medical conditions.

There are many variables that straightforwardly influence the strength of every one of your organs and the degrees of synapses in your body and in this way impact your feelings. The following are a couple:

Supplement and lacks of nutrient, like vitamin B3, vitamin B6, vitamin B12, L-ascorbic acid, folic corrosive, zinc, fundamental unsaturated fats (EFAs), and different supplements that influence emotional wellness.

Horrible eating routines, like such a large number of straightforward carbs and sugars or too little protein and vegetables. Lacking supplement ingestion due to a failing stomach related framework.

Food bigotries and sensitivities.

How much activity you do. Customary activity lessens misery and uneasiness by expanding synapses in your body and expanding oxygenation of your cerebrum and your organs.

Glucose balance. Shaky glucose frequently causes sensations of tension or gloom, particularly when insufficient sugar takes care of your cerebrum.

Hormonal lopsided characteristics brought about by outer estrogens, contraception pills, and water poisonousness.

Ecological and weighty metal harmfulness like lead, copper, mercury, aluminum, pesticides, and compound poisonousness.

In the forthcoming parts, you will figure out how to cure these variables and recapture control of your physical and profound prosperity.

WHAT IS ANXIETY AND DEPRESSION?

"Very much like the inconspicuous flows make winds, which you can feel, which move a leaf, which you can see, so do inconspicuous contemplations make feelings, which you can feel, which make illness or recuperating, which you can see. We are all nature… "

I Abhorrence Utilizing the word melancholy since it has such a weighty and extremely durable feel to it, and it accompanies its own disgrace. The word gloom doesn't appear to assist anybody with moving past their profound state and here and there makes individuals feel more regrettable when they are named with it. I like to say it's anything but an answer situated mark. Personal trouble is a superior word since it seems more like a brief circumstance, so I use it conversely with the words tension and sadness.

Sadness, uneasiness, and other dysfunctional behaviors are analyzed by specialists as per the Demonstrative and Measurable Manual of Mental Issues (DSMV). In this manual, various marks are given to various psychological circumstances, contingent upon the side effects an individual has and on the power and recurrence of these side effects. Names given to individuals incorporate despondency nervousness over the top- urgent turmoil, significant sorrow and occasional emotional issue, summed up nervousness jumble, distrustfulness, bipolar, schizophrenia, post-horrible pressure confusion, and others.

Comparable side effects do, obviously, exist across various marks. For instance, individuals with summed up nervousness confusion and significant despondency both experience side effects of uneasiness, albeit the recurrence and force of side effects in each mark contrast. Also, individuals with over the top enthusiastic problem and summed up tension turmoil both experience changing levels of suspicion and uneasiness, simply in various sums and with various coming about ways of behaving.

Despite the fact that different psychological circumstances are given various names, a significant number of them share comparative compound awkward nature. This similitude implies that unique temperament issues are really comparable cycles happening in the body with various triggers and various degrees of force. This being said, make an effort not to get genuinely connected to a determination that a specialist could give you. The main driver, the impacted organ framework and your uniqueness are more pertinent to your recuperation. By knowing these significant perspectives, treatment becomes less difficult and more successful.

For Jane's situation it is essential to understand that her side effects of uneasiness and discouragement are a consequence of her one of a kind reaction to a harmful dad and shaky home climate. Jane is not the same as some other individual, so the manner in which she answers pressure, diet, or ecological impacts is unique in relation to how others would respond in comparative conditions. It is likewise fundamental to comprehend that others with comparable feelings to Jane could have an alternate reason to their feelings and need an alternate way to deal with their treatment.

For instance, one more understanding of mine, Tina, 33 years of age, had endured from tension and sorrow since she was a youngster. Regardless of how much guiding she attempted, she didn't improve. We at long last figured out that she generally got restless and discouraged subsequent to eating wheat. Her stomach related framework was bigoted to gluten, a substance tracked down in wheat and different grains. The compound responses to gluten in her body were changing her mind science, prompting her sadness. In the wake of eliminating wheat from her eating routine, she recuperated totally!

<u>SYMPTOMS OF DEPRESSION AND ANXIETY</u>

An individual is determined to have discouragement commonly when they have five of the side effects underneath more often than not, enduring for longer than about fourteen days, and on the off chance that these side effects slow down their social or work life. I accept a large number of us endure with a portion of these side effects to the point of justifying recuperating, despite the fact that we probably won't be determined to have a psychological sickness.

- Extreme sensations of culpability, sadness, despair, as well as uselessness.
- Trouble concentrating or trouble deciding. Rest unsettling influences — either sleep deprivation or sleeping late. Pointless or persistent touchiness.
- Staying away from social circumstances and exercises or withdrawal from individuals. Weakness or feeling tired frequently for reasons unknown. Absence of inspiration, interest, or delight in exercises they used to appreciate.
- Sobbing oftentimes for reasons unknown, feeling miserable constantly, and acquiring no joy from anything.
- Loss of or expanded hunger or weight. Successive considerations of self-destruction.

Ordinary indications of nervousness include:

- Alarm, anxiety, hyper-excitement, dread, neurosis, and meddlesome or undesirable contemplations.
- Vulnerability, trepidation, hesitation, sadness, or feeling incapacitated.
- Consistent concern, pressure, uneasiness, or uncomfortable sentiments that have not an obvious reason.
- Failure to have positive expectations about overseeing straightforward circumstances.
- In some cases wretchedness and uneasiness might appear with actual signs, for example,
- Free defecations, looseness of the bowels, stomach issues, or queasiness
- Troublesome or shallow breathing, snugness in the chest, heart
- Palpitations, sensations of faintness, discombobulating, dry mouth, or sweat-soaked hands.
- Muscle torments, jaw snugness, grating teeth around evening time or during the day, absence of rest, or ongoing weariness.
- Various circumstances that could cause tension in individuals include:
- Being in parties.
- At the point when an individual is let be and is awkward being separated from everyone else.
- At the point when glucose levels drop excessively low, because of physiological issues like hypoglycemic episodes.
- At the point when somebody is gone up against with their fears; for instance, fizzling a test, meeting individuals, seeing a canine, or being presented to levels.
- At the point when somebody is helped to remember a horrendous encounter that has not been completely settled. This is most frequently found in post-horrendous pressure problem (PTSD).

Various individuals answer contrastingly to comparable circumstances, which is the reason each individual should be dealt with extraordinarily and independently. The way an individual shows their side effects, be it uneasiness, gloom, or neurosis, relies upon their one of a kind qualities, including hereditary qualities, diet, and physical and profound cosmetics. An individual's day to day environments, work and social feelings of anxiety, support frameworks from individuals and local area programs, financial status, and other factors additionally influence their capacity to adapt to pressure and influence the way their feelings create.

MENTAL ACTIVITIES TO FURTHER DEVELOP PROSPERITY AND RECUPERATE THE PAST

"A man excessively occupied to deal with his wellbeing resembles a specialist excessively occupied to deal with his instruments."

A Base Piece OF your mind, known as your limbic cerebrum, is intended to safeguard you through instinctual endurance systems. Your limbic cerebrum responds consequently to circumstances in light of past upsetting encounters you have had, and it can keep on acting in a protective mode despite the fact that the underlying compromising experience may as of now not be available in your life. In the event that a horrible or unpleasant experience isn't completely settled, your cerebrum will unknowingly keep on conveying distressing messages to your body, particularly your adrenal organs. These signs put pointless and delayed weight on your body, unavoidably prompting adrenal weariness, sickness and close to home issues.

Psychotherapy, profound opportunity procedure, homeopathic meds, and different treatments that I depict underneath assist with liberating your cerebrum from its oblivious focused on state and return it to its loose or unbiased state, which likewise stops the pressure your brain puts on your adrenal organs. Mending unpleasant close to home recollections really changes unfortunate brain associations in your cerebrum into better associations, utilizing brain adaptability, which is the capacity of your mind to rework its nerve associations. Such changes really modify the profound understandings you have of old distressing recollections, permitting you to have more sure feelings and a more drawn out enduring better viewpoint on life.

The practices in this section assist your cerebrum with settling distressing circumstances from your past. They permit your cerebrum to supplant pessimistic or distressing feelings with better feelings and thought designs utilizing brain adaptability. This leaves you less damaged and less focused than previously. As you do these activities, make sure to diminish aggravation and recuperate your body too, as I have depicted to some degree 2 of this book. Aggravation and unequal chemicals

(If it's not too much trouble, see Section 2) really decrease the capacity of your cerebrum to make better nerve associations, causing it challenging to feel genuinely well regardless of whether you attempt and stay good through these activities.

Everyday act of these activities will diminish your inclination to stretch, tension, despondency, and negative considerations. Your brain will start to have a real sense of reassurance.

At the point when your brain has a good sense of reassurance, you start to unwind and turn out to be more open to more joyful sentiments feels more prepared to do as such. Having a positive and loosened up mind likewise makes a difference you to expect more sure encounters in your day to day existence, which significantly has an impact on the way you move toward life and carries better things to you. Your general bliss will in this manner be more a consequence of the inside recuperating of your own discernments and feelings, as opposed to changes of outside conditions in your day to day existence.

Every one of these activities should be possible independently or together, and some should be possible consistently. I profoundly propose doing every single activity and doing the day to day ones consistently. Attempt and do each activity subsequent to perusing it as opposed to going through them in your brain. You need to completely participate in these practices for your psyche to encounter their total advantage.

DEVELOPING EMOTIONAL RESILIENCE

The accompanying activities are things you can do every day to foster a positive outlook and better profound flexibility. Use them routinely, particularly when you are going through troublesome times, and watch out for change!

What Went Well the Earlier Day

Research shows that recollecting and recording what worked out positively for you during the day the builds your satisfaction for longer timeframes. I generally do this practice in the mornings in bed, particularly when I used to awaken with that horrendous feeling of fear, hopelessness, and despair. Recollecting and getting on paper positive encounters assists your cerebrum with bettering recognize that positive encounters are genuinely a piece of your life and that not much needs to change in your life for you to feel great consistently. Composing and zeroing in on sure encounters consistently likewise breaks your example of encountering negative considerations and convictions, what's more, you will ultimately understand that you can feel much better more often than not.

By the day's end and each day when you awaken, intellectually go through or record what you achieved or what worked out positively for you during the day and the earlier day. It very well may be completing a responsibility, figuring out how to work out, going out with a companion, triumphing ultimately, or in any event, getting a grin from somebody.

Ensure you recognize something like eight conditions that worked out positively for you or on the other hand that satisfied you. Attempt it now. Endure 20 minutes recording everything that worked out positively or didn't turn out badly for you for the beyond 2 days. I've left some space for you here to do this:

GIVING YOURSELF PERMISSION TO HEAL

A ton of our intense subject matters really come from an oblivious opposition we need to permit ourselves to acknowledge a superior approach to being. A significant number of us are too reluctant to relinquish specific thoughts or feelings we have become used to. You probably won't actually know about these inconspicuous protections which keep you away from feeling significantly improved. I have made an activity which permits you to conquer some of these oblivious protections. I utilized this exercise effectively while working with survivors of the Kenya Westgate fear monger assault, and, even after such a horrible experience, I saw individuals' uneasiness strip away, their breathing change, what's more, their injury and strain go to a murmur and grin of help. It's a very strong activity whenever done well.

I'd like you to begin an everyday work-out where you share with yourself: "it's protected to (… be blissful, have this impression, let go, mend, major areas of strength for feel, in affection, and so on…)" Or "it's OK to

…" and feel what occurs within you as a portion of your restricting contemplations start to surface. This is a strong activity you can do at whatever point you feel any close to home uneasiness. I've utilized it ordinarily and am constantly shocked to find what contemplations have been keeping me down without me in any event, knowing it.

At the point when you attempt this activity, scan inside yourself for what you might want to feel or what you're battling with, and say "It's protected to… "Add "at times" or "sometimes" after your sentence. This assists your psyche with tolerating your sentences significantly more without any problem.

Regardless of whether you feel something negative and you don't have any idea what conviction is keeping you down, take a stab at saying "It's protected to feel as such and recuperate" you'll unexpectedly allow yourself to relinquish your inner turmoil and feel a liberating sensation and interior strength. I'm posting a couple of sentences to help you on your way.

Notice how you feel subsequent to expressing every one of these sentences. In the event that you feel any opposition or feeling coming up, acknowledge these sentiments and permit them to change as you contemplate further on your good expectation.

"It's protected (alright) to feel OK here and there." "It's protected (OK) to be content once more."

"It's protected (alright) to be rich and fruitful now and again."

"It's protected (alright) to be good with these sentiments once in a while."

"It's protected (OK) to be enamored once more or to adore somebody again at times." "It's protected (alright) to be in power once more."

"It's protected (OK) to have affection toward myself again every so often." "It's protected (OK) to feel as such in some cases."

"It's protected (OK) to grin to myself again every so often." "It's protected to feel significant once more, on occasion."

"It's protected to cherish myself once more, now and again."

<u>BEING APPRECIATIVE</u>

I used to battle with what being thankful means. I assumed I was being thankful in light of the fact that I wasn't actually censuring anything throughout everyday life. I felt that in my sub-conscience I should currently be appreciative. Nonetheless, after a couple of enlightenments of acknowledgment in my life, I started to understand that being thankful is about completely and effectively valuing explicit sentiments and insights regarding individuals, things or occasions. Being appreciative includes a full hearted affirmation as opposed to something you assume you as of now would toward the rear of your care. Being thankful doesn't remove valuable time from significant things throughout everyday life however gives you back significant chance to feel what's truly valuable in your life.

Being thankful is a strong method for working on your close to home prosperity. Studies show that individuals who practice appreciation are less anxious and less discouraged. On the off chance that you at any point get up in the first part of the day with nervousness or a feeling of fear, go through some minutes feeling appreciation for however much you can, and go through everything that worked out positively for you, didn't turn out badly or made you grin or unwind the past day. Consistently record ten things you are thankful for. At the point when you awaken in the morning, say thank you for this superb day, and say thank you for in any event five things you are or can be thankful for. Scan your brain for individuals you could have expressed gratitude toward. Assuming somebody has been thoughtful to you previously, say thanks to them verbally

or on the other hand to you on the off chance that you can't snag them, regardless of whether it has been some time since you saw them last.

Rather than contemplating what isn't working out positively in your life or what you still

haven't achieved, ponder to what lengths you went for some of things you presently have and recognize that they are currently in your life, and feel a debt of gratitude.

Indeed, even in the most troublesome conditions, where nothing useful is evident, find something you can be thankful for, regardless of whether it inconsequential to the troublesome circumstance. Looking for positive parts of tough spots changes the way you answer life and gives you the fortitude to be more proactive and make more sure changes for yourself. Rehearsing this consistently will implant your psyche with positive contemplations and feelings so you are more outlandish to slip by into pessimistic sentiments.

Commit to yourself for the following 7 days to just envision what is working out positively or what worked out positively, doing this over the course of the day for 7 days, no matter what is happening. On the off chance that you're focused on or there's an upsetting circumstance, stop

briefly, and redirect your brain to contemplate what you are thankful for or what went well the earlier day, or what has been working out in a good way for you in your life. It very well may be straightforward things like "I have a bed to rest on", "I'm procuring some cash", "I'm thankful for my breath", or "I have a family or individuals who care about me". Over the long run your brain will naturally have more certain contemplations to contemplate, and will get away from distressing considerations and agonizing feelings. Go on now and expound on 10 things you can be thankful for in the space I've left for you:

SETTING POSITIVE INTENTIONS

"To wish to be well is a piece of turning out to be well."

In some cases when we need change in our life, we center a lot on the negative thing we need to dispose of. All things being equal, discuss what you need in a positive way.

State what you need, which gives your brain and heart a reasonable expectation to work on, as opposed to expressing out loud whatever you need to dispose of, which is seriously griping about your circumstance and building up your pessimistic considerations and sentiments. For model, as opposed to say, "I need to dispose of my bitterness and misery," say words like, "I need to feel more joyful in my life." The subsequent sentence expands the sensation of what you need in you, and it makes you more mindful of the means involved to get you to where you need to be. It additionally makes you mindful of certain sentiments or thoughts that you have and were not ready to abandon. This clearness expands your capacity to do whatever it takes to bring positive changes into your life. Compose no less than ten positive change sentences for yourself, and read them without holding back no less than one time per day or while you're feeling desolate.

Here are some certain change sentences that will assist you with beginning:

- ➢ I need to feel more settled in my life (as opposed to saying, "I need to feel less restless.")
- ➢ I need to grin more regularly.
- ➢ I need to have more sure considerations
- ➢ I need to be and feel blissful. I need to chuckle more.
- ➢ I need to be seeing someone is blissful and congratulations.
- ➢ I need to be where I feel free and cheerful. I need to have positive contemplations about what's in store.
- ➢ I need to feel revived in the first part of the day. I need to feel monetarily free.
- ➢ I need to be more joyful with myself; I need to contemplate myself and grin.
- ➢ I need to feel sure about myself. I need to mend from this.

Be explicit about your objectives and wants. Feel free to record some on paper. Push yourself, investigate, appreciate, and truly feel the things you need! Initially, it may be challenging to nail down unequivocally what you need; in any case, as you do this process, a feeling of clearness will arise, and it will be more straightforward to envision what really encourages you. Inevitably, you will naturally start to relinquish trouble, despair, and other pessimistic idea examples, and you will actually want to zero in additional on sure contemplations and feelings.

EFFECTIVE MEDITATIONS

"Nature, time and persistence are three incredible doctors."

There was a period in my life when I was very worried, confounded and hesitant and had no clue of what I genuinely needed for myself. I went to various specialists, and they generally helped a little, however nothing halted the disarray or gave me a feeling of harmony until I began to ponder. As straightforward as it sounds, it was one of the most remarkable gifts I gave myself. It assisted me with interfacing with an internal truth that truly felt like my own, and this gave me such a lot of force resist the urge to panic, make my own choices and comprehend what I truly needed for myself.

The vast majority have their own particular approach to contemplating; be that as it may, certain individuals find it very hard to ponder. I have depicted a couple of basic procedures for you beneath. Rather than attempting to reflect for quite a while at one sitting, it is more remedial to do more limited reflections habitually during the day, in any event, for just five minutes all at once. Reflection assists you with growing more positive considerations and pursue more levelheaded choices for yourself. Everyday contemplation further develops synapse levels in your mind, decreases nervousness, lifts your mind-set, assists with settling further intense subject matters, and associates you to your higher profound self.

A Simple meditation

Sit in an agreeable position either on a pad on the floor, or on a seat, with your back straight and the backs of your palms laying on your thighs.

Contact the tips of your thumbs to your pointers. Shut your eyes delicately, and shift your brain's concentration to your breathing, permitting your breath to follow its regular musicality.

Envision that your breath is made of white light and love, and this light and love is saturating each cell of your body and mending all aspects of you any place it goes, including your contemplations and feelings.

Reflect in a quiet, clean, and cleaned up climate, ideally near certain plants or out in nature. Share your recuperating light and love with the plants around you and envision the plants offering their mending light and love to you. This expands how much sure energy you get from the climate.

Contemplate for something like two minutes whenever you get an opportunity during the day, and afterward leisurely move gradually as long as ten minutes or longer.

Assuming that your psyche becomes swarmed with contemplations during your reflection, notice these contemplations without attempting to battle them away and without passing judgment on them. As you notice these contemplations, see what responses they bring out in you, and permit those responses to happen without battling against them. Allow these contemplations to vanish delicately as you get back to your representation. Permitting your considerations and sentiments to go back and forth during your reflection creates agreement and persistence to you and assists you with turning out to be more agreeable and certain in yourself. As you become more alright with your sentiments, your considerations will have less ability to make pressure in your body.

Different types of contemplation, aside from zeroing in on your breath, incorporate picturing various pictures, like brilliant light in the middle of your brow, a quiet candle fire, the sea, the sky, or nature.

One more method for contemplating is to imagine words like satisfaction, love, pardoning, and harmony. Grinning and reflecting on sure words can very inspire. Shut your eyes and envision the word euphoria, and let your sentiments follow bliss. Grin when you make sure to grin and loosen up in the impression of bliss.

Thinking day to day makes amicability in your heart, and you will feel less upset by distressing circumstances. Energy will come all the more normally to you, and you will start to feel more OK with yourself.

FORGIVENESS, FRUSTRATIONS AND EXPECTATIONS

Pardoning can be something troublesome some of the time. The vast majority of us, in any event, when we attempt to excuse, are still left with a sensation of harmed or disillusionment. This is typical.

Despite the fact that you realize it very well may be great for you to pardon somebody or something, your psyche probably won't be prepared to give up or neglect. Once in a while, truth be told saying "I excuse you" to somebody actually leaves you with an inclination that something wrong occurred among you and that the individual could in any case be liable.

Through my preparation in family heavenly bodies' treatment, I viewed as a new modest and more complete approach to saying "I pardon you". It's by saying "Please accept my apologies this occurred for me with you", or "Please accept my apologies this occurred for us", or "Please accept my apologies this occurred for me with us", or a comparative variant to this. Saying it along these lines permits you to acknowledge and relinquish what is happening all the more totally and calmly.

It likewise eliminates any fault you actually hold for the individual and doesn't leave you with a misguided feeling of predominance. Give it a shot. Regardless of whether you want to pardon somebody who hurt you or frustrated you, have a go at saying this, either to them straightforwardly or to you, and see what occurs. Absolution liberates your brain of negative energy, considerations and fault. It permits you to push ahead more calmly and emphatically.

Hatred and frustration torture your psyche, make you more negative\ furthermore, and keep you from carrying on with life decidedly. Essentially, neglected assumptions can be an extraordinary wellspring of oblivious burdensome energy that we haul around with us.

As indicated by certain advisors, neglected assumptions and frustrations, particularly connected with our folks, can be a wellspring of persistent sadness without us knowing it. Ponder all the neglected assumptions or frustrations you have encountered with individuals. Whether you anticipated that they should work on something for

you, or on the other hand on the off chance that they acted with a specific goal in mind, or then again assuming they took something from you - anything that it is, do a psychological check and check whether you have any outrage, disdain, frustration or miserable sentiments around any recollections. Presently, truly let go of these assumptions and disillusionments, and say the pardoning sentence "Please accept my apologies this occurred… "To these recollections. Truly put forth a psychological attempt to pull away from this stale energy which is keeping you away from carrying on with life and grinning to yourself frequently enough. Say "It's protected to give up", or "It's protected to feel along these lines", or "It's protected to feel pardoning here and there", or some other sentence will free you from the grasp of disdain and disillusionment. When you can get away from these sentiments, your mind will revamp itself, and you will let loose some psychological space for additional good contemplations and sentiments.

EMOTIONAL FREEDOM TECHNIQUE

Created by Gary Craig, Close to home Opportunity Strategy (EFT) is one of the quickest developing strategies individuals are utilizing to track down alleviation from profound issues. In EFT, you express articulations about your sentiments and tap on specific needle therapy focuses on your body. Despite the fact that EFT might appear unusual to do from the start, EFT brings huge close to home alleviation right away and changes negative convictions and insights into additional positive encounters.

To perform EFT, pick an inclination or experience you are battling with and that you need to change into a surer one.

Utilizing your right fingertips, tap on the plump piece of the edge of your left palm underneath your little finger (known as the "karate hack point") while saying the accompanying expression multiple times: "Despite the fact that I… (Say your issue here, e.g., "am wounded by my accomplice's egotism toward me" or "am feeling truly discouraged at this moment"), I profoundly and totally love and acknowledge and regard myself."

Abbreviate your beginning sentence into a rundown sentence (for instance, the above sentence can turn into, "hurt by Steven's haughtiness"), and tap no less than multiple times on the accompanying focuses on your body while saying the abbreviated variant of your sentence:

1. On the bone close to the inward corner of your eyebrow (left or right eye, it doesn't make any difference)
2. On the bone on the external edge of your eye
3. On the bone under your eye
4. On the tissue over your lip and under your nose
5. On the tissue over your jaw and underneath your lower lip
6. On the internal piece of your collar bone
7. On your fourth rib under your bosom
8. On your ribs under your armpit

You could feel a change in mindfulness about your sentiments, and you can modify your sentence to match your new sentiments. For instance, you could say "less discouraged" or "feeling significantly better" while you keep on tapping. When you come to the end tapping point under your armpit, begin once more in the event that you actually have any gloomy sentiments left.

Change your sentence to match any new sentiments intently you are encountering. This is an improved on variant of EFT and more subtleties and more exact tapping focuses can be tracked down on the web, including free manuals on EFT. The magnificence of EFT is that it utilizes needle therapy focuses as well as certain confirmations to make new brain associations in your cerebrum, and it releases close to home brief delays, making long haul benefits without any problem.

<u>HEALING RUMINATION</u>

"Now and again your bliss is the wellspring of your grin, yet some of the time your grin can be the wellspring of your delight."

Rumination happens when you invest energy contemplating your issues, self-reflect adversely, center around sentiments related with negative circumstances in your life, or ponder how you could have done things another way.

Rumination frequently includes different considerations like apprehension, stress, lament, culpability, and disgrace, which re not arrangement situated or forward-moving. Rumination stresses your mind and aggravates nervousness, and it likewise keeps you from taking part in better considerations, discussions, connections, and exercises that would keep away from pessimistic sentiments. Unfortunately, focused, restless, tired, and discouraged individuals find it harder than others to stop rumination furthermore, transform their considerations into additional positive ones, making this an endless loop.

Rumination happens when your psyche has not or can't completely determine a troublesome profound encounter. Guiding, particularly psychotherapy, decreases rumination by assisting you with dealing with profound encounters. By discussing your thoughts with a specialist and delivering troublesome feelings, your cerebrum makes new brain associations that are less genuinely charged. . This mending permits you to feel more joyful and have better considerations.

Rumination is here and there difficult to defeat since it includes manners of thinking that are attempting to tackle significant issues in your day to day existence. Regardless of whether you need to stop, you could have a restless outlook on relinquishing rumination since it implies you will leave your concern strange and leave yourself defenseless against the tough spot. Feeling sufficiently great to relinquish rumination and spotlight on other charming things will accompany practice.

On the off chance that advising isn't a possibility for you, there is one more method for beating rumination. To start with, you want to perceive that rumination increments mental pressure and melancholy and doesn't address a lot. Second, contemplate the things you commonly ruminate on and recognize circumstances or times when you generally ruminate (like heading to work, sitting alone at home in the nights, and so forth.). Discover yourself ruminating each time it works out, and track down an interruption quickly. The following are a couple of ways you can break the rumination cycle.

Telephone a companion, pay attention to some music, play with your pet, or go shopping and take part in discussions with the shop's staff or even with an outsider. In the event that you would be able, discuss your thoughts with a companion since it assists with getting an alternate point of view on your concerns and potential arrangements.

Do the wide range of various activities portrayed in this section. Lay out an image or diary about your viewpoints by expounding constantly on them for five minutes in a row without taking your pen off the paper. Free writing in this manner discharges feelings and makes better brain pathways in your cerebrum. By resetting brain processes, your cerebrum loses a portion of its inclination to ruminate on similar recollections in light of the fact that you have changed the profound setting of the recollections through the close to home release.

Begin saying positive insistences constantly. Positive assertions break the pattern of negative idea designs and furthermore help you to start accepting that you can feel alright. When you start trusting in more sure conceivable outcomes, your brain turns out to be more persuaded and you wind up feeling better on a more regular basis. Express things to yourself like: "I'm cheerful, fortunate, solid and favored"; "beneficial things happen to me each day"; "life is getting endlessly better for me consistently"; "I feel better inside"; "Feeling as such"; "I love you (to yourself in the is OK"; reflect)"; "You mean a lot (to yourself in the mirror)"; "some of the time these things occur and it's alright"; "sympathetic myself is OK here and there". Regardless of whether you can't accept or feel the substance of these sentences right now, keep saying them in light of the fact that by centering on sure certifications rather than negative ruminating considerations, your mind really feels less worried and gradually starts to overhaul itself towards better wellbeing.

Do a speedy arrangement of sit-ups or push-ups; run on the spot; clean the dishes; record how you really want to help the week; go for a speedy walk; or reflect on sure contemplations like love, harmony, and euphoria. I view practice as one of the most incredible ways of breaking rumination, particularly while I'm practicing with another person. Having organization, regardless of whether you converse with one another, assists you with drawing in with another person as opposed to being distracted and segregated with your own contemplations.

I try not to eat alone however much as could reasonably be expected. Eating alone can be incredibly discouraging. Assuming that you must be separated from everyone else while eating, pay attention to music or work on being thankful for each easily overlooked detail in your life, including each nibble of food. Concentrates on show being thankful reliably limits the movement of despondency. At the point when I was visiting

India, an inn really had a goldfish swimming in a bowl on each table involved by single individuals.

Do whatever isn't contemplating your issues, regardless of whether it implies painting, grinning at the mists, conversing with a tree, or snickering at yourself.

COMPLETING SMALL TASKS

Time and again in discouragement we leave our life wrecked and permit incomplete exercises to rot. A discouraged individual isn't inspired to do a lot. The incomplete errands wait to us and go through a great deal of oblivious energy. We lose energy along these lines, and hesitation becomes both a propensity and a battle. The issue is, the more undertakings you leave incomplete, the seriously overpowering your life is by all accounts, deterring you more from attempting to achieve anything and discouraging you much further.

By achieving little undertakings like cleaning your room, covering a bill, keeping in touch with one email, or taking your canine for a walk, your psyche really feels a feeling of achievement, fulfillment, and delight. Regular encounters of achievement, delight, and fulfillment reinforce your feeling of certainty also, inspiration, empowering you to effortlessly do different assignments more. On the off chance that you're feeling stuck, simply believe that you need to get done with one little responsibility, and regardless of how unmotivated you feel about it, and invest in finishing it. Keep in mind, it could be essentially as little as mailing a letter, tidying up your room, taking care of a bill, composing your objectives for the week (a great action), or calling somebody you love.

When you begin feeling the fulfillment of little achievements and perceive hesitation as the aversion of gambling with change, you will feel inspired to do something else for your life. Simply start with each errand in turn, at the present time!

HEALING THE PAST

The following arrangement of activities help to let old and existing injury out of your psyche so you can let loose your brain to turn out to be more present and appreciate life all the more completely. Make an effort not to re-damage yourself when you think about a portion of your old recollections - be delicate with yourself and look for proficient assistance in the event that a portion of these recollections are too challenging to even consider managing all alone.

Timetable Delivery Recuperating Journal

Here and there getting a general viewpoint of our encounters in life assists with recuperating a great deal of our convictions and sentiments. In this activity, I'd like you to draw a timetable diagram of your life, starting from birth till your current life. You can utilize the diagram I've drawn for you. On the left side, as indicated by time, list all the physical encounters that altogether affected you. On the right side, list all the profound encounters you have had in your life that either caused you to feel embarrassed, damaged, pushed, liable, unfortunate, or undesirable, or made some other it was awkward to feel that. Regardless of whether you feel these encounters are unessential for you today, record them still, since when they happened, they had an effect on you, but little.

Presently, beginning with the latest profound experience, expound ceaselessly on anything that strikes a chord encompassing your experience. Compose for fifteen minutes without taking your pen off the paper. Keep composing regardless of whether what you're composing doesn't check out. This exercise assists you with delivering caught feelings associated with your encounters and assists you with seeing your life all the more plainly and tranquilly. Do this for a limit of two previous encounters each day, not more, since you won't completely determine the encounters in the event that you swarm your psyche with a ton of profound handling.

You could have to rehash this activity for specific occasions that take more time to determine. Take as much time as is needed in this mending venture. Show restraint toward yourself. Try not to decide your message on paper. Simply keep composing throughout the following couple of weeks or months and notice how much better you feel as you get a reestablished and more enabled point of view over your life.

Relaxed Breath in Past Memories

This is an activity I made and find that it functions admirably. On the off chance that you have any memory that is unpleasant or negative, I welcome you to reconnect with that memory to you. As you envision yourself in that particular situation, notice how you are relaxing. Start quieting your breath down, taking in a casual way as you still spotlight on the memory. Permit your psyche and feelings to move as you keep on quieting your breath down. Trust simultaneously and acknowledge whatever changes are occurring. Utilize this activity on each experience you have composed down in your course of events recuperating journal and notice how different you feel. Indeed however this appears to be an exceptionally straightforward activity, I find it extremely valuable in aiding our mind revamp a portion of the upsetting recollections that we convey.

Changing Your Story

Throughout everyday life, we frequently make a story for ourselves. For instance, you could make statements like, "I haven't recuperated since my better half said a final farewell to me," or "I feel exploited by what occurred, and it was unreasonable," or "I was too modest as a youngster so I never made an adequate number of companions at school," or some other story that you continue to distinguish yourself with. In the event that you distinguish yourself with what I call misled or feeble stories, you consistently act as though these accounts actually meaningfully affect you, and it becomes challenging to make better and more useful ways of behaving until you start to change your account of yourself.

In the event that you retell your story to yourself and to others another way, actually keeping it honest, you allow your cerebrum an opportunity to change and to feel a feeling of control over the circumstance as opposed to feeling misled. I tell you, this is one of the most remarkable and extraordinary activities I have encountered.

For instance, a little story from my life as a youngster could be retold in the accompanying way:

My educator approached me one day in the study hall and was exceptionally cross that I had my lunch box close to my work area. I had no clue about that this was an issue. She gotten it and flung it across the floor to the opposite finish of the homeroom and shouted at me. I felt outrageous disgrace and fear and have feared her of all time since.

I can dial back the occasions in my memory into various pieces, making it simpler for my cerebrum to deal with little pieces of the story in little advances:

I was perched by my work area when unexpectedly my educator approached my work area and resented me for something. I'm not exactly certain what. In her displeasure, she got my lunch box and tossed it across the floor. I was embarrassed and confounded, and I think it was on the grounds that my lunch box was close to me, despite the fact that I am as yet not certain assuming this was the genuine issue.

Since I have isolated various pieces of the experience into discrete close to home parts, I can see plainly that maybe the educator was not just furious with me, however an irate individual. I might in fact attempt a little humor in my story to make it lighter for me:

My educator was a truly severe and irate lady, and every one of the children feared her. She even came dependent upon me one day and tossed my lunch box across the floor of the homeroom and shouted at me. I was stunned, and every one of the children were astonished, yet we realized that was her normal way of behaving.

In retelling the story this time, I understand that a ton of children feared her and that perhaps she was a for the most part irate lady. I allow myself an opportunity to feel less culpability and disgrace about the entire circumstance since every one of the children feared her, also, her displeasure was not just customized toward me. I out of nowhere feel a feeling of support from every one of the children in the study hall. Maybe my educator didn't have the foggiest idea how to act fittingly with youngsters and was sincerely flippant. As I understand the consensus of my educator's outrage, I feel a slight change in my body where I was clutching some trepidation from before, and I presently feel less undermined by the memory of her.

It could take many endeavors for you to feel less sincerely impacted by your story. This is completely fine. Each time you feel a slight change in mindfulness or feeling, your cerebrum is recuperating from the occasion. You can likewise work your story out in an unexpected way commonly and go through the mindfulness shifts all alone; nonetheless, it's better to do it with individuals as a result of the lively trade you get from offering to individuals. You can likewise do this collectively of around at least five individuals, with every individual blending with various individuals in the gathering, retelling their story in various ways with every individual. Work on changing one of your recollections beneath, multiple times, and check whether it has an effect on you:

Envisioning Positive Encounters

One more activity to determine close to home injury from an occasion is to envision the occasion happening on a phase or on a TV screen, with you as an observer in the crowd. As you watch the experience, envision the occasion happening somewhat in an unexpected way. Utilize your brain to acquire helping scenes or more sure results to the occasion.

For instance, to recuperate myself of a circumstance when I was genuinely manhandled by somebody from quite a while ago, I envision him on the screen turning away momentarily from me and being keen on something different. This reduces the force of his glare and really assists me with breathing somewhat more profoundly. As I proceed with the activity over the long haul, I may be prepared to envision this individual leaving occasionally. This gives me more breathing space and assists my cerebrum with going back over the occasion in a more loosened up manner. Doing this more than once really reworks your cerebrum and modifies your feelings encompassing unpleasant recollections, hence preventing your mind from persistently focusing on your adrenal organs.

Another memory I recuperated this way is the point at which I found it hard to recuperate from the extraordinary pain I went through during a drawn out separation with my better half. It was a significant stretch of dismissals and contentions where I endured a lot. How I reduced the power of my pain was to envision her on the screen grinning at me sometimes during our difficult situations. Doing this diminished the aggravation in my psyche that was still there and assisted me with grinning a bit, as well. I didn't have to change the whole memory — I adjusted it unpretentiously enough so it stayed credible to me. As I proceeded with this activity, I really settled a ton of melancholy and confidence gives that originated from this occasion and figured out how to foster a sound connection with another person.

A third model is the memory of a truly mean educator to me when I was a kid. As I imagine him on the screen glaring and yelling at the little me,

I envision a bird stopping on his shoulder. Naturally, this releases the concentration in my mind from his annoyance and threatening shift focus over to something else delicate and protected to encounter for a small kid. I could try and envision my folks or on the other hand someone bigger coming to converse with him as an approach to safeguarding me. This too lessens the nervousness in my oblivious memory. Since I'm less compromised also, feel more secure sincerely with my memory, my mind quits sending upsetting oblivious signs to my adrenal organs, and I recover a portion of my close to home strength.

You could at first feel extraordinary feelings doing these activities. As you proceed to do them, the force will reduce in light of the fact that your cerebrum will have released a portion of the pressure related with your recollections. Adverse occasions from quite a while ago ruin your realness and change the manner in which you act with others. If you keep on carrying on with your life in a repaid way, you sustain the negative sentiments you convey within you. As you recuperate genuinely from previous occasions, you start to feel more certain and open in your life. Recuperating is an open door to stir a more liberated and more blissful self and to cooperate with the world in a more sure and self-strong manner, which will ideally bring you better wellbeing and more certain encounters.

Ho'oponopono

Ho'oponopono is an old Hawaiian act of excusing and cherishing the part within you that is encountering an injury or upsetting occasion. Ho'oponopono became renowned when Dr. Ihaleakala Slash Len in Hawaii restored deranged lawbreakers without seeing them. He would concentrate on their clinical graphs and search inside himself to find what portion of his cognizance made the individual's sickness in his world. As he pardoned and cherished this part inside him, Dr. Len figured out how to fix an entire ward of patients.

This appears to be an implausible story, but it has worked for some individuals and is in light of the rules that everybody's reality is a projection of what's within them and we are liable for all that we experience in our reality. We can mend anything by getting a sense of ownership with the experience and mending the part in us that is making the experience. To do Ho'oponopono, at the point when you feel upset by a circumstance or have a previous injury that isn't completely mended, permit yourself to open up to the part within you which feels hurt or upset by the experience, whether it's previously or in the present. When you feel this spot within you, place two hands over your heart region in the middle of your chest and say the accompanying words to this focused on piece of you with as much love and empathy as could really be expected:

"Please accept my apologies, I love you, I excuse you, much obliged."

You can imagine these words quietly, murmur them or express them without holding back. Continue to express them to the focused on part within you, notice how you feel and trust the progressions you are feeling inside. Do Ho'oponopono on each experience you wrote in your course of events mending journal to assist with diminishing the feelings encompassing tough spots in your day to day existence. I do Ho'oponopono on day to day circumstances and on many previous encounters and I frequently notice a change in my feelings, in the manner in which I connect with individuals and in the manner I act now.

Chipping in

Did you had at least some idea that chipping in for a worthwhile motivation really works on profound prosperity?

Indeed, it's valid. I've done it without anyone's help various times and it truly feels great. Concentrates on show that chipping in really mitigates melancholy and forestalls individuals from backsliding into melancholy too. Chipping in likewise helps you foster interactive abilities, allows you an opportunity to make contacts and companions, and forestalls social separation, which is a significant reason and result of despondency.

Chipping in is in many cases peaceful and can feel fulfilling, meaning your body will all things considered produce endorphins (warm hearted chemicals) from feeling fulfilled and appreciated. Give your chance to a genuine goal this end of the week, or at whatever point you have available energy. Face a challenge and figure out what may be a good time for you to do. Really you don't need to place yourself in a tough spot to chip in - I spent one end of the week establishing trees on Mount Kenya for the sake of preservation. I'll have food to a halfway house for youngsters with Helps each Sunday, which is a truly pleasant thing to do in light of the fact that the giggling and embraces from the kids feels so great. These are only several instances of decent conditions where you can volunteer your time. Also, who knows, you could try and assist somebody with evolving their life for the better with a novel gift you didn't actually acknowledge you have!

FRIENDS, FAMILY, AND SUPPORT GROUPS

"Companions are the medication of life"

Opening up to and acquiring support from family, companions, and self-improvement gatherings can have a major effect on the off chance that you experience the ill effects of intense subject matters. It very well may be threatening from the beginning, however unveiling your concerns to a dependable individual beginnings a chain response of help and profound delivery. They could offer you guidance, share a comparative circumstance in their lives, or know somebody who can help you. Regardless of whether you don't get all the assist you with requiring from the primary individual you converse with, sharing your concerns with one individual gives you the boldness to open up and look for further assistance with others.

As a companion or relative of somebody with intense subject matters, it is significant to listen cautiously when the person uncovers sentiments and not be critical. Show that you give it a second thought and are keen on the issues instead of promptly attempting to propose arrangements. An individual uncovering nerves and intense subject matters is being open to you. The more you tune in and permit that individual to feel alright sharing this weak side, the more grounded and more open to assist the individual in question with willing turn into.

Ask how you can be of help, yet attempt to be patient and nonjudgmental if your assistance is declined. Individuals with personal challenges frequently struggle with judging the best arrangement. Another way you can help is to track down contemplation, yoga, individual development, or self-improvement gatherings. Maybe you can go to a couple of meetings with the individual to give some consolation. Having support at the underlying gathering or request assists disintegrate numerous hindrances with peopling experience while first looking for help.

www.ingramcontent.com/pod-product-compliance
Lightning Source LLC
Chambersburg PA
CBHW050818250726
48653CB00006B/2303